MAKING THE ASSIST

CARING FOR THOSE WITH CANCER

MAKING THE ASSIST

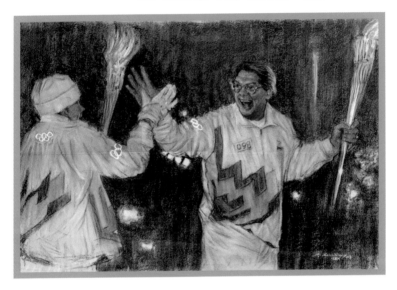

CARING FOR THOSE WITH CANCER

J. David Pitcher, Jr., MD

With contributions from
H. Thomas Temple, MD, Sue Heffelfinger
Michael Spafford, MD, and Ingrid Sharon, MD
Illustrated by L. Henry (Hank) Jones

VIP
VISION IMPRINTS PUBLISHING
A Thomas Nelson Company

www.thomasnelson.com
Tulsa, Oklahoma

MAKING THE ASSIST
Copyright © 2006 J. David Pitcher, Jr., MD

Published by Vision Imprints Publishing
A Thomas Nelson Company
8801 S. Yale, Suite 410
Tulsa, OK 74137
(918) 493-1718

ISBN: 1-599519-12-X

Library of Congress catalog card number: 2006920035

Printed in Singapore

What Others Are Saying . . .

This book teaches through personal experiences and anecdotal tools that to deal with the possible loss of life, the most important ability is being able to trust and love God. I recommend the reading of this humble and instructive book as a source of daily inspiration to anybody who is involved either professionally or personally in the care of people with cancer.

Reza J. Mehran, MD
Associate Professor, Thoracic Oncologic Surgeon
University of New Mexico Cancer Research and
Treatment Center
Albuquerque, NM

Making the Assist is like a game plan to coach family members of loved ones with cancer. It motivates us to not guard our feelings, to not stand on the sideline, but to move forward in being involved.

Kimberly A. Dean, DO
Family Practice
Largo, FL

My friend and colleage, Dr. David Pitcher, has written a valuable guide to those who are caring for friends and family with cancer. I have seen how cancer affects the lives not only of my patients but also of their loved ones. These are often the overlooked victims of the disease. This book gives them strength, comfort, and encouragement.

Gregory Fotieo, MD
Internal Medicine
New Mexico VA Health Care System
Albuquerque, NM

Dr. Pitcher, a respected orthopaedic oncologic surgeon and the author of this book, helps the caregivers of patients with cancer in performing a most challenging and demanding task with fortitude and courage. He has drawn from his faith and personal experience, examples that give hope where otherwise despair and hopelessness could reign.

Mohinder Mital, MD
Orthopaedic Surgeon
Albuquerque, NM

Dedicated to my mother and father who showed me on their own courts that the best shot is to serve.

I lift up my eyes to the hills—where does my help come from? My help comes from the Lord, the Maker of heaven and earth.
Psalm 121:1-2

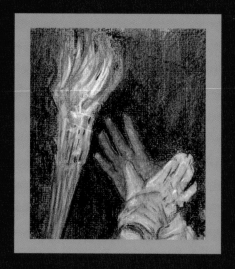

It is one of the most beautiful compensations of this life that no man can sincerely try to help another without helping himself.
Ralph Waldo Emerson

Contents

INTRODUCTION

Not Forgetting to Pick up a Jersey

by Michael Spafford, MD
Head and Neck Oncologic Surgeon
Albuquerque, New Mexico

"You can give without loving,
but you cannot love without giving."
Amy Carmichael

❖   ❖   ❖

*The chapters of your life
involve other people.*

God is our refuge and strength,
an ever-present help in trouble.
Therefore we will not fear, though
the earth give way and the mountains
fall into the heart of the sea, though
its waters roar and foam and the
mountains quake with their surging.
Psalm 46:1-2

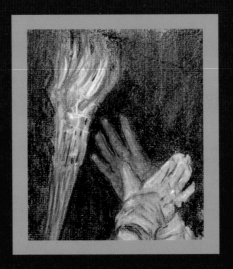

There is nothing, no circumstance,
no trouble, no testing that can ever
touch me until, first of all, it has come
past God and past Christ, right
through to me. If it has come that far,
it has come with a great purpose.

Not Looking at the Camera

*The longest part of the journey is said
to be the passing of the gate.*

Marcus Terentius Varro

You cannot get involved until you take that first step.

In this you greatly rejoice, though now for a little while you may have had to suffer grief in all kinds of trials. These have come so that your faith—of greater worth than gold, which perishes even though refined by fire—may be proved genuine and may result in praise, glory and honor when Jesus Christ is revealed.
1 Peter 1:7-8

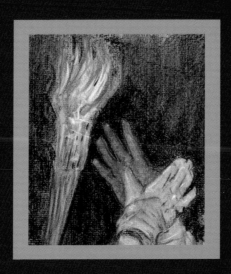

When God permits His children to go through the furnace, He keeps His eye on the clock and His hand on the thermostat. His loving heart knows how much and how long.
Warren Wiersbe

Not Losing Heart

by H. Thomas Temple, MD
Orthopaedic Oncologic Surgeon
Miami, Florida

*Hope does not lie in a way out,
but in a way through.*
Robert Frost

In a time when physicians care too much about financial reimbursement and medical malpractice, it is refreshing to reflect on this series of vignettes by the author, Dr. David Pitcher, who underscores the importance of caring for others. He has recognized the inherent good in being able to "facilitate" the success in others. To "make the assist," he points out, is his satisfying asset. This is a book about caring. It is also a book about encouragement and hope. Giving unto others and being fulfilled in that act.

As physicians, especially surgeons, we must realize that there is a fundamental difference between curing and healing. Curing requires wisdom and skill. Wisdom is needed to recognize the problem and to know what to do. Skill is essential to act on that wisdom. The process of healing on the other hand, is divine providence and results in fulfillment for those who participate in the process. Healing however does not always result in curing.

As Dr. Pitcher points out, there are certain diseases that are incurable despite extraordinary wisdom and great skill possessed by those who treat these maladies. But though there is no cure, healing may supervene. Anyone who treats and cares for those with cancer can affirm this. As the author quotes Beard, "when it is dark, you can see the stars." No one knows this better than Job when he says, *"If only my anguish could be weighed and all my misery be placed on the scales! It would surely outweigh the sand in the seas"* (Job 6:2-3).

We are all subject to God's merciful will. Everyone, including the "greatest and least amongst us." The author implores us to cure when we can, but to care deeply always. That we should follow God's own example of caring found in John 3:16, *"For God so loved the world that He gave His one and only Son."*

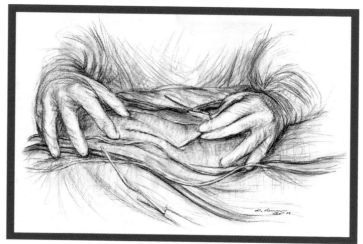

Dr. Pitcher is an orthopaedic oncologic surgeon, a surgical specialist that treats bone and soft tissue cancers. Ironically, during the course of his training to become an orthopaedic oncologist, his beloved cousin tragically died of a rare bone cancer called osteosarcoma.

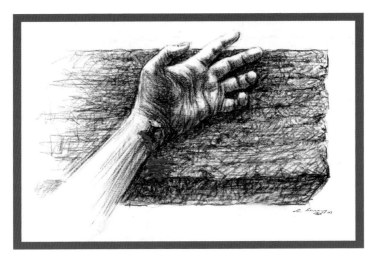

He, as many of us have experienced at one time or another, missed an opportunity to be involved in the life and inevitable death of a loved one, an experience that leaves an emptiness and irreconcilable void. He points out that we do get distracted, consumed by our own troubles, and sidetracked from our primary mission, that of caring. To avoid this, he offers strategies to stay involved despite these distractions and encourages us to find fulfillment in service unto others and importantly, to not get discouraged—to "stay the course."

The wise and skillful can cure but by the grace of God, only the caring can participate in healing. This is the profound, powerful, and simple message, one that should resonate amongst all who are truly blessed to attend to those in need.

Only those who care
can truly participate in healing.

*Even youths grow tired and weary,
and young men stumble and fall;
but those who hope in the Lord will
renew their strength. They will soar
on wings like eagles; they will run
and not grow weary, they will
walk and not be faint.*
Isaiah 40:30-31

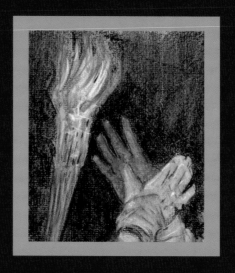

*The big question is whether you are
going to be able to say a hearty yes
to your adventure.*
Joseph Campbell

ACKNOWLEDGEMENTS

Not Neglecting to Get Started

with Sue Heffelfinger
Caregiver, Albuquerque, New Mexico

Over every mountain there is a path,
although it may not be seen from the valley.
James Rogers

I'd like to thank all my friends and family members who have reviewed this manuscript and have made suggestions. To my bride and love, Pam, and to my family, I wish to acknowledge that, without them, I would not know what to give. And to my Lord and God, I acknowledge I would have nothing to give, without Him. A friend of our family, Sue Heffelfinger says it best when she quotes Billy Graham:

> *"He will give us strength*
> *when we have none of our own,*
> *courage when we are cowardly,*
> *and comfort when we are hurting."*

I asked Sue to help me put this into words because of her first hand experiences in "making the assist." We saw her put many of the aspects of her life on hold while she helped her husband. She wrote, "My husband Steve was diagnosed with Hodgkin's lymphoma in November 2001. He completed his course of treatment, which included chemotherapy and radiation, in May of 2002. This was the first time that cancer had touched either of our families. We were determined to put our confidence in God, knowing that beyond a shadow of a doubt Steve's life was and still is, in God's hands. '. . . *let us run with perseverance the race marked out for us. Let us fix our eyes on Jesus, the author and perfecter of our faith, who for the joy set before him endured the cross, scorning its shame, and sat down at the right hand of the throne of God. Consider him who endured such opposition from sinful men, so that you will not grow weary and lose heart'"* (Hebrews 12:1-3).

She continued, "Are you weary, are you losing heart? There is one who wants to carry your burden and be your support and strength . . . He is even 'more faithful than a brother' and His name is Jesus. When I could hardly turn on the engine of my car to go to work, He was there to strengthen me. In the wee hours of the morning when I wondered if we would still be together in a year, Jesus reminded me that He has gone before us to prepare a place for us in Heaven . . . for eternity where there would be no more pain and no more tears. He reminded me that I could keep a quiet heart. Even now, as we face the unknown, the Lord has said to me, 'Hush, and be still. . . . Do not be afraid any longer, only believe.' As a caregiver, you will need to be cared for as well. Search your heart. God offers peace and hope to all through His Son, Jesus. All you need to do is open the door of your heart and ask Jesus to come in and He will meet you right where you are. He alone has been my strength and peace. I would like to share a verse from the Bible that has been the anchor for my soul during this time: '. . . *I know whom I have believed, and am convinced that He is able to guard what I have entrusted to Him for that day'"* (2 Timothy 1:12).

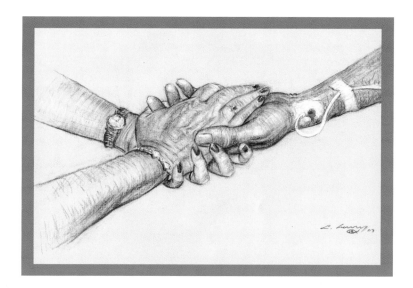

The place to start is the acknowledgements. Acknowledge that you cannot do it alone. You need a team. You need other family members and friends, and you need a coach, Almighty God, and His game plan, His Word, the Bible. Acknowledge that the care and love in your heart is a quality given to you by God. Take the words and thoughts from this book and let them *paint* their way into your words and thoughts. It is my desire for you, that this book, *Making the Assist*, will encourage you in your getting into His game plan for this season of your life.

You must acknowledge that you cannot get involved solely relying on your own strength.

. . . He said to me, "My grace is sufficient for you, for my power is made perfect in weakness." Therefore I will boast all the more gladly about my weaknesses, so that Christ's power may rest on me. That is why, for Christ's sake, I delight in weaknesses, in insults, in hardships, in persecutions, in difficulties. For when I am weak, then I am strong.
2 Corinthians 12:9-10

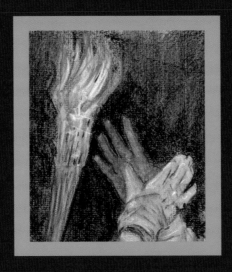

Tried for a season, pure for eternity.
Warren Wiersbe

Not Forgetting to Pick up a Jersey

by Michael Spafford, MD
Head and Neck Oncologic Surgeon
Albuquerque, New Mexico

*If we had no winter,
the spring would not be so pleasant;
if we did not sometimes taste of adversity,
prosperity would not be so welcome.*
Anne Bradstreet

If you have picked up this book, chances are that someone you love has been diagnosed with cancer. Together you are beginning a journey into the unknown, and it is terrifying and overwhelming. Know that one in seven persons in developed countries will start out on the same road this year. For most of you this is completely uncharted territory, but not for Dr. David Pitcher. With his friendly, intelligent, and cheerful manner he has guided many people, young and old, through this forbidding terrain. They have found that by taking small steps they were able to manage each obstacle. Having this book in your hand demonstrates your commitment to your loved one. Reading this book is one of the small steps that will help you to manage well what has been placed before you.

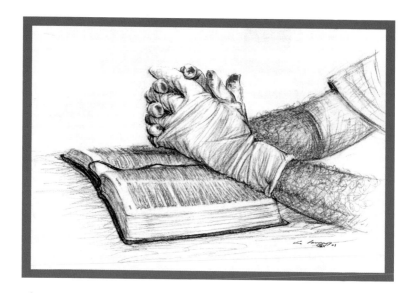

As Dr. Pitcher explains, this is a chance to live fully, although the culture in which we live may imply otherwise. Serious illness and even death are things that we will all experience. If we are fortunate, we will love and be loved through these times. Just as what normally happens through marriage or the birth of a child, caring for one facing illness and death takes us deeper into the all-out, sold-out, radical commitment to one another for which we are purposed. We are *designed* to love one another.

> *"Place me like a seal over your heart, like a seal on your arm; for love is as strong as death . . ."*
> Song of Songs 8:6

This kind of love, possible in our everyday human relationships, points to a greater reality which is too important to miss. In the following pages you will be reminded of One who dealt squarely with our weakness, illness, and death and felt that His own life was not too great a price to pay. It is He who will lead you on this journey.

Only those who love can truly care to participate in healing.

The Lord your God is with you, he is mighty to save. He will take great delight in you, he will quiet you with his love, he will rejoice over you with singing.
Zephaniah 3:17

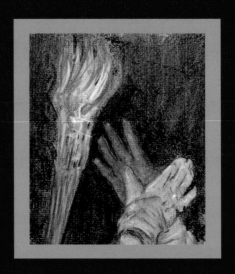

Those who navigate little streams and shallow creeks, know but little of the God of tempests; but those who "do business in great waters" these see His "wonders in the deep." Among the huge Atlantic waves of bereavement, poverty, temptation, and reproach, we learn the power of Jehovah, because we feel the littleness of man.
Charles Spurgeon

CHAPTER ONE

Not Having a Say-So

*You are here in order to enable the world
to live more amply, with greater vision,
with a finer spirit of hope and achievement.
You are here to enrich the world, and you
impoverish yourself if you forfeit the errand.*
Woodrow Wilson

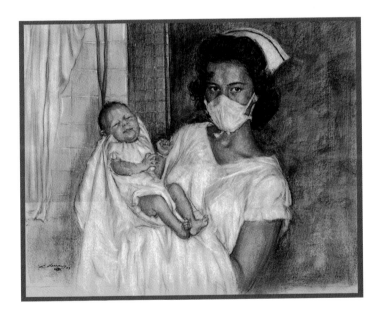

I was born the middle child between two girls. The first recorded picture of me is not in my mother's arms like my two sisters, but in the arms of a nurse. You see, I was born breech, and the delivery was very difficult. My mother was not in any shape to hold me like she did with my two sisters. I was delivered with forceps and the obstetrician had to put a bone hook into my sternum to pull me out. I have a scar at the top of my sternum where the bone hook went in. I guess that was my first introduction to medicine. It was also my first introduction to service. Although I did not know it at the time, my mother put herself at risk for me. I was not able to speak out against such a risky procedure. I had no say-so.

Such is the situation that many find themselves in today. A loved one has been diagnosed with the possibility of losing their life to a malignancy. The uncertainty of chemotherapy, the thought of radiation therapy. Placed between two options, to get involved or to hide in isolation. Yet all the time, held in the arms of a loving God who wants to introduce us to an unconditional love. A risky procedure, and we have no say-so as to whether He offers it to us or not. He already has. And this is the love that can sustain us and help us to choose involvement and not isolation.

Many years ago, I sat down and looked at all the elements in my life and discovered the common thread. This common thread formed the basis of the purpose of my life. Everybody's purpose is different, but mine is "to facilitate the success of others. To make the assist." Whether it is playing second violin in an orchestra, helping our kids get through college, teaching orthopaedic surgery, or treating patients with musculoskeletal tumors, I'm a helper, a facilitator. And I'd like to help you through a time that you don't understand, that I don't understand. A time when a loved one of yours has been diagnosed with the possibility of losing his or her life from a malignant tumor, from cancer. *This moment may be the most important moment in your life.*

Looking back on my life, it seems that I have been molded by the Potter to accomplish the task set before me. Although I don't always do the task perfectly, when I am in His hands, He makes this cracked jar of clay hold water. He can do the same for you in the most difficult task of helping someone with cancer. I like Jeremiah 18:3-4 where God is in control of molding a person's life. *"Then I went down to the potter's house, and there he was, making something on the wheel. But the vessel that he was making of clay was spoiled in the hand of the potter; so he remade it into another vessel, as it pleased the potter to make."* If you will let God take your life and use it for another, it will be pleasing to Him.

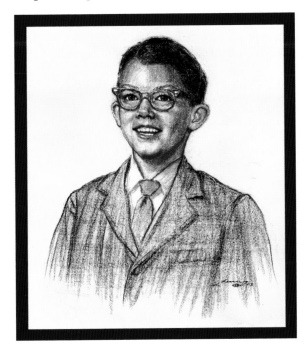

You may not have a say-so in being placed into the situation of helping someone with cancer, but you do have a say-so in whether to help the person. The journey will not be easy, but it will be rewarding, and will leave a lasting mark upon your life and upon your legacy. It will stretch across a generation to the next. It will not be forgotten. But to get involved for the reward is to go at it for the wrong reason. You must have a heart for it.

I am not writing this book because I think I am qualified. Certainly there are those who have made it their life message to help the persons around them who have cancer. There are those who are in volunteer organizations and even those who are paid. You will see from my life that I have been at fault for not being involved myself, but I have also reaped the benefits of helping those with cancer. It has been and continues to be a harvest in my life of inconceivable worth.

Two older books on this subject are *Don't Waste Your Sorrows* by Paul E. Billheimer (Christian Literature Crusade, Fort Washington, PA, 1977), and *Does My Father Know I'm Hurt?* by Doctor David John Seel (Tyndale House Publishers, Wheaton, IL, 1971). Some of my favorite newer books are *A Window To Heaven* by Doctor Diane M. Komp (Zondervan Publishing House, Grand Rapids, MI, 1992), *When God and Cancer Meet*, by Lynn Eib (Tyndale House Publisher, Inc., Wheaton, IL, 2002), and *A Bend in the Road* by David Jeremiah (W Publishing Group, Nashville, TN, 2000). Find other sources that will help and encourage you. Study God's Word on subjects such as encouragement and hope.

Please learn from my mistakes. You would think that as a physician and surgeon I would have not been so slow. You can't do it from within yourself. The greatest lesson that I have learned is that God decided when time began to get involved in my and your life. He has shown us the reason for getting involved and what it is that can sustain us during the days of chemotherapy, radiation, or surgery. What is it that we can pass on to our loved ones during the most important time of their lives? Sacrificially giving our love. *Your whole life, like mine, has brought us to this point.* We are ready for the challenge!

Your involvement must come from love for another.

Greater love has no one than this, that he lay down his life for his friends.
John 15:13

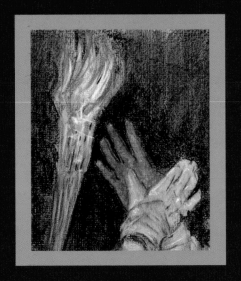

The greatest good you can do for another is not just share your riches, but to reveal to them their own.
Benjamin Disraeli

CHAPTER TWO

Not Being the First Draft

I want to be thoroughly used up when I die.
For the harder I work the more I live.
George Bernard Shaw

I had just become a teenager when my grandmother, Anna Karban Wyatt, "Grammy," came and lived with us for a short while after having been diagnosed with breast cancer. She didn't live very long, but I remember the time my mother spent taking her to doctor's appointments and to church services. Times have changed and the life expectancy of a person with cancer has lengthened since the 1960s. For example, a person with osteosarcoma had less than a 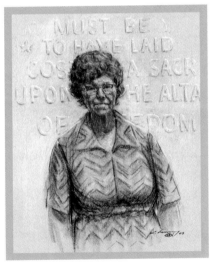 20 percent chance of living over five years. Now, with effective chemotherapy, that number is approaching 80 percent. Other malignancies have a similar change in prognosis. This puts an ever increasing burden on the person who steps up to help another with cancer.

We had a three bedroom house at 4640 South Delaware in Tulsa, Oklahoma, that was situated at the bottom of a cul-de-sac. The old land maps showed that it was situated in the middle of a dry creek bed. Every time it rained, water flowed into the back of the house through a sliding glass door soaking the carpet. It was a big deal to have my grandmother live in our home. All of our family laid down sacrifices. It was a period of growth for me that I would have not obtained otherwise. Perhaps you feel flooded. Perhaps your involvement will influence only your life. Most likely, your commitment to love another will go far beyond your life.

I wasn't a particularly popular boy at school. I didn't excel in sports or in any particular ability. I couldn't win simultaneous chess matches with the first violinist and second violinist next to me, making moves during the rests of *My Fair Lady* or whatever we were practicing at the time. Although I thoroughly enjoyed wood shop and usually made an A on my projects, I wasn't the best in the class. I even was number thirteen on my peewee baseball team, the "Oilers," because that was the only number that was left.

I delivered papers on my "Stingray" for the *Tulsa World*. I prided myself on being able to ride up the hill from the drop off service station where we folded, rubber banded, and packed papers into bike baskets and front and back canvas packs. One icy morning just after 5 AM, I was hardly going up the hill when the tires slipped on the road and the papers spilled all over 51st street. It was too large a load, and I had to walk the bike for the first couple of apartment buildings until the load lightened. Perhaps you feel your load is too large.

That is sometimes the situation we find ourselves in throughout life. Our baskets are too full. It's OK to walk the bike or to ask for help. It's OK to leave some of the load for a second trip. It's OK to play second violin, or to sit on the bench and guard the water bottles. The net effect of my delivering papers was that after a year, I had saved up one hundred dollars and could buy a ten-speed Schwinn bicycle. That bike could fly! I could get from our house to my grandparents' house at 1826 East 16th Place in less than thirty minutes, a distance of over four miles.

On one day back, I decided that I could ride with my hands crossed. I could easily ride without hands, so I reasoned that I could simply put my hands on the handlebars and . . . hit the pavement! No sooner than I put my hands on the handlebars that I hit the road flying at full speed. Bruised and scraped, I twisted the handlebars back into alignment, and satisfied that no one had witnessed my clumsiness, I got back into the saddle. Perhaps you feel thrown from the saddle of your routine.

When I graduated from high school, my grandfather, Edgar Roy Pitcher, "Pappy," wrote me a letter which began "My Dear David." One of the things he wrote was "May knowledge bring you a great measure of humility and always remember that there are many things more to learn." There is no way for me or another person to prepare you for the road ahead of you. It is a road you must walk with a great measure of humility. You must learn many things. You must learn the width and depth and breadth and length of love, and that your love will last. . . .

❖   ❖   ❖

Your love will last far beyond your own years.

Now I know that the Lord saves his anointed; he answers him from his holy heaven with the saving power of his right hand. Some trust in chariots and some in horses, but we trust in the name of the Lord our God.
Psalm 20:6-7

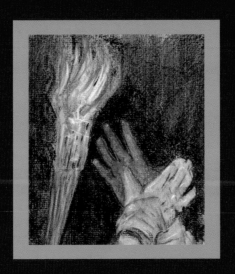

Thus would I double my life's fading space; For he that runs it well, runs twice his race.
Abraham Cowley

CHAPTER THREE

Not Making the Rules

The value of life lies not in the length of days,
but in the use you make of them . . .
Michel de Montaigne

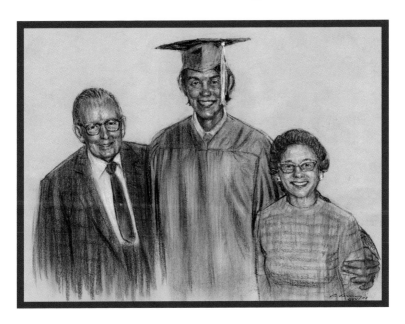

My grandfather, "Pappy," was diagnosed with lung cancer when I was in college. I loved him dearly, but I had not really known him well. He had a great compost pile in the back of his garage and there were always worms for fishing. That compost pile took a lot of time to turn over and water, but the net affect was a beautiful backyard garden with roses, gladioluses, irises, and vegetables. What a wonderful experience for a youngster. I prayed that he would live long enough to know that I would see him again someday in heaven. When I asked him, he taught me about his love for his Savior.

Talk about the things that matter most with your loved one. These are the things that will strengthen both of you. No matter what the age of the person, there are important things to talk about. It seems that teenagers are the hardest to open up. They are ones with often the most profound things to say. Getting their hopes and fears out on the table won't make them easier to face, but will allow you both to face them together.

Be honest and sincere. The word sincere comes from two Latin words which mean "without wax." If a pot had a crack in it, wax was often put in the cracks and this would hide its uselessness from the unaware buyer. The emphasis is not on the uselessness of the vessel, but on the deception on the part of the seller. Maybe you feel useless in this situation. You will be very useful if you remain open and honest, even if you are "cracked" and only able to hold a little water.

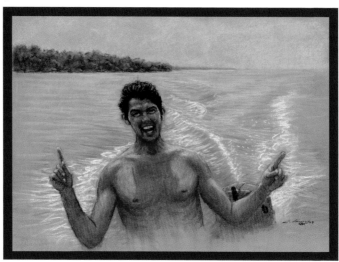

During one of the summers between college semesters, my dad and I, and another father and son navigated the Verdigris River from the Port of Catoosa in Oklahoma to another port in Arkansas. This is the kind of time it takes to be open to another. Use the time you have together to talk about likes and dislikes, lessons learned and lessons forgotten. Learn from one another of the grace of God.

Get on the person's own eye level and make eye contact. Follow their eyes with yours, their emotions with yours. While being trained in orthopaedic oncologic surgery, I noticed patients who had been seen by one of my professors, Doctor Henry J. Mankin, often thank him for spending so much time with them. He actually spent very little time with most patients because of his busy practice at Massachusetts General Hospital in Boston, but made it seem so by putting the patient completely at ease by getting comfortable and at their level.

Don't seem to be in a rush. Make the person feel as though they are the most important person in the world right now, because in fact, they are! Your job, if you choose to accept it, is not an impossible mission at all. Your job is to impart the love in your heart to another. It's that simple. There's no other rule or hidden agenda.

> ❖   ❖   ❖
>
> *Your love will surpass*
> *the rules of life and death.*

*Be imitators of God, therefore, as dearly
loved children and live a life of love,
just as Christ loved us and gave
himself for us as a fragrant offering
and sacrifice to God.*
Ephesians 5:1-2

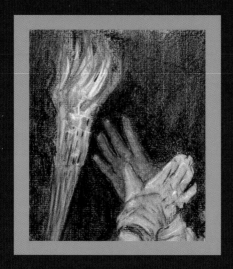

*It is only with the heart that one
can see rightly; what is essential
is invisible to the eye.*
Antoine de Saint-Exupéry

CHAPTER FOUR

Not Getting the Top Contract

We are made for cooperation, like feet,
like hands, like eyelids, like the rows of the
upper and lower teeth.
Marcus Aurelius

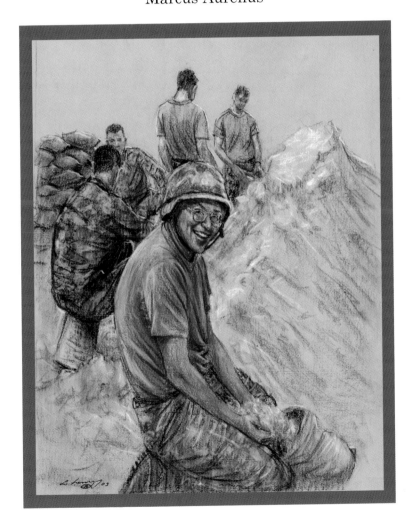

There I was, filling sandbags at Fort Polk, Louisiana. An orthopaedic oncologic surgeon, doing my field time. A bit outside the operating room. Certainly outside my environment. Perhaps you can relate. You are helping a person with cancer. In some ways you are extremely over qualified. In other ways you are not. Whatever your chosen profession, this experience is going to help you grow, and have an influence on others that you can't imagine and would never expect. It won't be comfortable, but if you roll up your sleeves, the bags will get filled.

There are many uses of sandbags. Holding back flood waters, weighing down road signs, and stacked around tents are some of the uses. They are all meant for protection. And that is your role. You are a sandbag for the person with cancer. Protection against discouragement, against loneliness, against hopelessness. Without your involvement, the person will likely fail.

I never enjoyed going out into the "field." I was an eagle scout, but that was different! There was the time we awoke to machine gun fire and we had to make our way to the PT boats to evade the "enemy." I dropped my 35mm camera in the river . . . Or how about the time we spent in a bunker in mosquito infested Panama over Easter? Or how about the times of deployment to Wuerzberg over Christmas and New Years? Having to sleep in our gas masks and chemical warfare suits. Think beyond your box. Get an award winning photo with medics "made over" with bloody moulage in a Panama bunker.

Bring your wife over for a surprise New Years in a German castle. Play the violin while in the gas mask! Thinking beyond yourself is a start to getting the most out of the "contract" you have been given and making it into a "covenant."

There are many other things you could be doing right now. Some of them need your attention right now! This is one of those things. It's time to put aside the other chapters in your life and let this one take precedence. You will never forget the experience, nor will you ever be the same. Moment for moment, caring for one who has cancer is the most rewarding experience you will ever have. Giving of yourself without hope of gain, without the possibility of return, will give you a joy from within that cannot be gained elsewhere. The emotions you will feel, the tears you will shed, will be greater than any motion picture or soap opera. They will be the real thing. This will be real living. This will be a real sacrifice.

You say it is impossible! And so it is. No one can give of himself without the well eventually running dry. There must be a Source of your giving. "They say" that you can't take "it" with you. But this is part of your life that you can take with you! And you will influence others while you do it selflessly. It will take courage and perseverance on your part. Are you up to the task? There is not another who could take your place!

Perhaps there is another "soldier" who can help your friend or loved one along side of you. You don't have to do it alone! But you must get involved! Develop a network of friends who can help your friend or loved one beat this disease called cancer. No one can do it alone. Your pay will not be measured in dollar amounts. The appreciation may only be in a tightly held hand, in a frightened hug, in a glance of the eye. Rest assured, this payment will be enough. It will outlast all the other accounts you have in your name. But you must have yet another account from which to draw.

Your love must come from beyond yourself.

And Jonathan made a covenant with David because he loved him as himself. Jonathan took off the robe he was wearing and gave it to David, along with his tunic, and even his sword, his bow and his belt.
1 Samuel 18:3-4

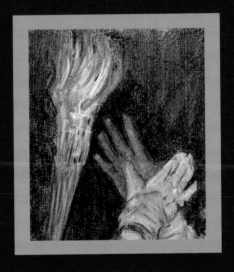

The longer I live, the more I realize that the greatest pain is often the place of greatest growth.
Luci Shaw

CHAPTER FIVE

Not Skipping Practice

*When it is dark enough,
you can see the stars.*
Charles A. Beard

While living in Tacoma, I liked to leave the house early for work, driving from the views of Puget Sound and the snow-capped Olympic mountains, through the tunnel of Douglas firs that seemed to form a force field around our neighborhood, rounding a corner to find the gentle pink early dawn painting a picture in back of the majestic Mount Rainier in northwest Washington. I had the road to myself and when it wasn't raining, I had the top of our little Geo Tracker down and felt the breeze and the freshness of it all. I listened to *Kip in the Morning* playing the latest in Christian praise and worship music, turning it up to make it part of the sound of the breeze. I could get the very closest parking space, and while putting the top back up (for you never know when it's going to rain again in Washington, but you can count that it will be soon!), enjoy the morning star and the moon retreating from the daylight. No pressures. The orchestra has stopped playing and the choir's a cappella interlude echoes with me still feeling the last vibration of the song on the radio.

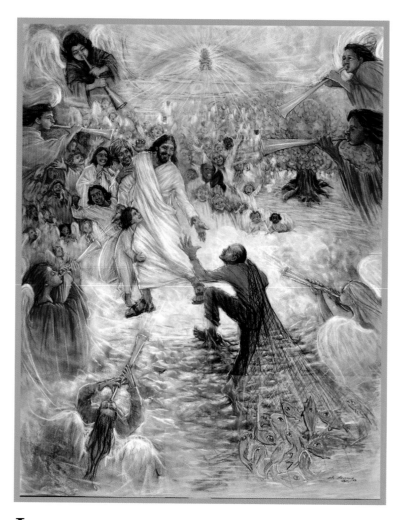

It's a calm that's out of this world. But this world always seems to get back into the picture with its turmoil. . . . Then it's into the side door of the clinic building and the usual chaotic schedule.

We have had our share of problems with all the drivers and the resources our devices use on our computer at home. Little technological problems seem to snowball. An awful warning will come on—BEEP—BEEP—BEEP—BEEP—and continues on and on until I press control—alternate—delete. The computer comes back on in safe mode allowing a self-diagnostic application to be used and find and correct the problem. You can push all the keys you want, but if you don't know how to get to safe mode the awful noise will keep blasting the calm from the day. One warning after another will appear on the screen causing the frustration and anxiety to mount.

Finding that calm Puget Sound that doesn't have a ripple on it really depends if you know how to do one thing: get into safe mode.

Let me help you find the way into safe mode for those days of turmoil (like today) so you can make the "practice." I had been running in it for about three weeks when my dad suddenly died after a heart valve operation. First it was a deserving applicant who wasn't selected for a residency position I thought he deserved. Then it was the agony of a thirteen year old patient with a malignancy in the lower leg bone clotting off her remaining vessel after I had removed the tumor to save her leg, watching her toes and foot turn black despite all of our best efforts to save her limb, ultimately resulting in an above knee amputation. Then the rejection of Jesus by two young people who failed to see the relevance of Him in everyday life. I felt like Job. I needed a friend and confided in a plastic surgeon and close buddy. Finally my dad died. November 15, 1996. I saw it coming. Fortunately, I was in safe mode. I think Dad was in it too. I had only learned to recognize it during the previous six months. He got there during his rare illness, Wegener's granulomatosis, leaving him dependent on renal dialysis for two years. Let me take you there.

Safe Mode Living

I have the distinct privilege of removing bone and soft tissue tumors, both benign and malignant, from patients. I have come to see that every single mother and father, when their child is afflicted by a limb or life threatening malignancy, would rather that they could take the place of the child. The pain, the suffering, even the death. I know this because they tell me. Directly and openly. Just after they ask, "Why?"

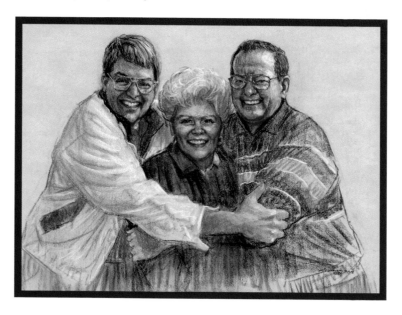

A mother's love. A father's love. It is obvious in my patients during their turmoil. It led me to the safe mode.

I was first introduced to Dutch ovens during Boy Scout campouts. There was still the *Old-Fashioned Dutch Oven Cookbook* in my room with recipes that included an *Expedition Mix* and *Hermit Cakes* at the time of my dad's death. Dad and I were both Eagle Scouts, and we have many memories of cooking on those outings. It was perhaps during one of those outings that I came to love cooking. I like to think it was the time when I used salt instead of sugar to make a peach cobbler. YUCK! Or maybe the time the cherry pie came out perfect, only to wind up upside down in the dirt by the fire. GRRR! Coals would be placed on top of the oven, and the cast iron pot would be set into the coals after the food to be cooked was placed inside. We've all had a Dutch oven kind of a day. A day when it feels as though the coals are below us, on top of us, all around.

All four Gospels record a day in the life of Jesus that was one of those Dutch oven days. There are only a few days in the life of Christ that all four Gospels record. Not even His birth is recorded by all of them. I think He wants us to know that He knows what we're going through when it happens to us. He knows exactly how we feel. *"For we have not an high priest which cannot be touched with the feeling of our infirmities, but was in all points tempted like as we are, yet without sin"* (Hebrews 4:15).

He knows how we feel when a family member and friend dies. John the Baptist, son of Elizabeth and Zechariah, knew Jesus as the Christ. He certainly was told by his mother how he leapt in the womb when Mary came to stay with his mother and her cousin. They certainly grew up together. Learned Scripture together. Experienced life together. He was probably His closest friend.

Then Jesus was told that John was dead. Not only dead but murdered, beheaded. Maybe you've lost someone and feel wronged for it; Jesus knows. It happened to Him. Not only that, but the very next thing Jesus learned was that Herod wanted to see Him also! *"And Herod said, John have I beheaded: but who is this, of whom I hear such things? And he desired to see him"* (Luke 9:9).

Find a Hideaway

What did Jesus do? He gets away for a while to a private place by boat.

My dad loved boats. He built, and to the day of his death it remained, a keel and struts of a large yacht in our garage. Unfinished. Begun in 1961. I found receipts for the ballast and other materials under his black socks in a folder labeled *boat*. A dreamboat. In fact, we called it our U.S.S. Dreamboat. In the months prior to his death, I think Dad accepted that the boat would never be completed by him. I think it happened the year before he died when I asked him where the plans were. We looked, but couldn't find them then, but subsequently found them. (I told my mom I'd like to finish it for him someday.) It was about that time that he started rejuvenating his fishing boat. He worked on the motor, the seats, and the trailer. He even built a shed by the side of the house under my old bedroom window to store it.

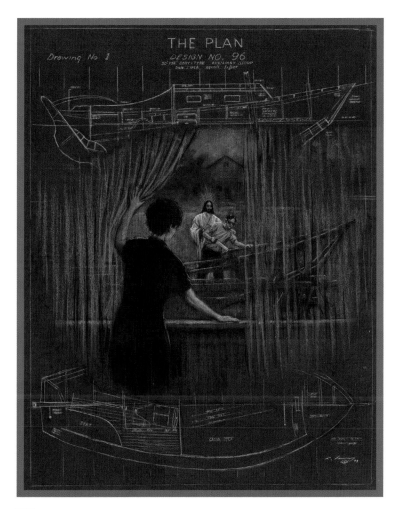

He loved *the country*. That was what we called Mom and Dad's little hideaway at Flint Ridge on the Illinois River near the Oklahoma-Arkansas border. When he had a problem that was way too big for him to handle, to our dismay, he was up at *the country*. He pulled through. Or maybe he was carried through. Find a hideaway. A private place. *The country*. A boat. A mountain. God will pull or carry you through. It may be only His footprints we see in the valleys,

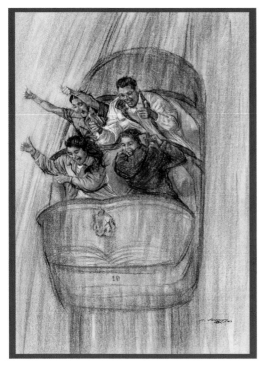

carrying us, when all other times He is there beside us, guiding, loving us.

Life is sometimes a roller coaster. Right before Dad was taken immediately back into the operative suite, because his infected aortic valve replacement was leaking, the doctors told us that everything went as well as could be expected. Dad had come off cardiopulmonary bypass like a champ (his coronary arteries were clear). Then he was whirled back in and later that night died. My sister Jo called me and simply said, "David, come home. Now. Daddy died." I was in Chicago with plans to be home later that day, having not heard about the return to the operating room. I had gone to sleep elated of the doctor's initial report. A *roller coaster* of a day.

Jesus knows. After the bad news of John's death, while He was in His private place, His disciples came and told Him of their stories of healings, deliverance, and teachings in His name. Ordinary guys made extraordinary by Him. On top of all that, five thousand men, not including women and children, found out where Jesus was and came to see Him. From the depths of sorrow to the height of seeing His friends succeed to the confusion of so many people.

Know the Worth of a Person in God's Eyes

Both Dad and I have degrees in medicine (*not really*). His is an *honorary degree* (from me!). He actually graduated from Tulsa University with a Bachelor of Science in Business Administration in 1956, the year I was born. He had kept, however, two comparative anatomy books that he had used. From his notes, that was a class and a half, maybe even a setback. Many setbacks occurred during his illness. Trying to get an arteriovenous fistula or AV shunt (as it is commonly called) to work was one of those setbacks. Many operative procedures were tried to get a mature shunt that could be used for dialysis. He always believed he would be healed and ultimately wouldn't need dialysis anymore. Constant checks were made on the status of these shunts. Since an artery and vein are connected, a little eddy current occurs at this junction in the blood stream which can be heard with a stethoscope. The noise is called a bruit—B R U I T (pronounced Bru' ey). He would always ask the nurse if anything was "brewing" in there.

Dad knew there wasn't any relationship between the words bruit and brewing except their sound. Still, it was his way of acknowledging someone who was helping him. Dad had long ago, during his forty-three years of selling office supplies for two companies, Scott-Rice and then Sooner Office Supply, found the worth of an individual. He had developed a way of looking at people and problems like our Master does. Know the worth of a person in God's eyes. He gets past the blemishes and pimples and sees our value. The value of you Rob, you Michael, you Crystal, you Aaron, you John, you Wayne, and you Rachel. Whatever your name. Dad always said that small companies would be able to compete with the big superstores because of one thing: super service. And being a super servant depends on one thing: realizing the true worth of an individual. Renal dialysis nurses and nephrologists were super servants to Dad.

They're not only super, but what they do is inconceivable! The kidney, with all its tubules and glomeruli, filtering all the impurities out of our system. To think, there is a machine that can do the job. Dad knew their worth you can be sure. It gave him a contagious meaning for the word inconceivable. It's inconceivable that I could fly in a vehicle that wouldn't even float. That I can get on the interstate and travel at 65 mph along with innumerable other people who are late picking their family up from the airport and not crash into their speeding missiles—inconceivable. That God would entrust to me two gems to help set into settings—inconceivable. That the sunrise on November 15, 2001, was an awesome array of reds and oranges for miles and miles—inconceivable. That the God who created the universe would write me a Book to tell me of His love for me—inconceivable. Those are the things my dad wants you to know. The worth of an individual is—inconceivable.

Talk with Jesus

He had his own opinion about medicine and healing. He had reviewed all the healings in the Bible. He accepted others' recommendations, but ultimately knew the glory would be God's. He, I know, shared his thoughts with Jesus. An ordinary guy made extraordinary by Jesus' presence. Talk with Jesus. Share your life, your intimate thoughts, your desires, and your victories with Jesus. He's been there. Experiencing it. He knows the ups. The downs. The ups and downs. Even when they occur back to back. When you don't know what to say to your friend or loved one, talk with Jesus.

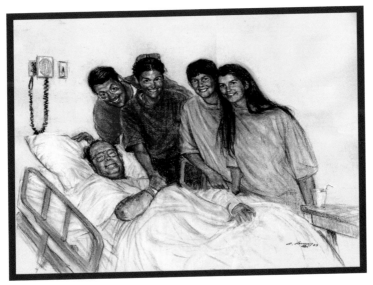

It was easy for Dad to hear God's voice. I'm not sure when it was that he began to hear it. After the Lay Witness Weekend at First Church in March of 1969, he began reading the Bible regularly. He had read about every version, taking a year to read and study each one. I can remember seeing him read his Bible during the lunch hour at Scott-Rice, where I worked during the college summer years. Our lives get so busy that we often put aside the important things and do the most urgent things. Dismiss the crowd like Jesus did, and get back to the mountain. Every day.

The disciples went across the sea of Galilee and you know the story. The wind was against them until Jesus came walking on the water. They hadn't learned from the feeding of the five thousand. Their hearts weren't open. They had expected Jesus to lead the multitude into Jerusalem and take His rightful position as King. He came to be the Sacrifice to pay the punishment for our sins. They hadn't dreamed of rowing back across the sea without Him. Jesus knew their hearts. What a letdown that must have been for Him.

I ran across a bunch of love letters that Mom and Dad wrote during their separation when Dad was with the Army. There must have been a hundred of them. I didn't actually read them. Fortunately, God's love letters to us are for everyone to read. And they are personal also. And that's how Dad was able to hear the Good Shepherd's voice.

". . . the sheep follow Him,
because they know His voice."
John 10:4

And in this very hour, the dad-sheep of our family still hears His voice.

Something tells me that Dad didn't resent his illness. It was a new experience for him to learn of God's grace and mercy, of His enduring love and everlasting peace. I never actually asked him that, but through it all I know he heard God's voice and finally kneels in His Presence. And we can learn from his experience. I know I have.

Say All Your Thank-yous

Don't forget to say thank you. The demands of life are all around us. Dad and I have both spent time in the Army. He made the rank of corporal, and I, a bit beyond that. Dad served two years with Headquarters and Headquarters Company, Third Battalion, 28th Division (from Camp Atterbury, Indiana, in Neu Ulm, Germany) during the Korean Conflict. Dad warned me not to "volunteer" for anything in the Army. Whatever it was that made him say that, he never said. I know it was something, because that's not what he did in life. If something needed fixing, Dad could and would fix it. His example must have rubbed off on me more than his warning.

Jesus saw those five thousand men and others coming and didn't say, "Go away, my best buddy just has been murdered." Hardly. He had compassion on them. He even fed them. And He stopped in the middle of it all, looked up to heaven and gave thanks.

You're going to say that it was easy to have compassion on them because He is God. That's certainly true. But He also knew everything about those people. There certainly were people who had done evil things among that number and those who wouldn't even say "thank you." He still had compassion.

Dad and Mom, thank you for showing me the love of God. Thank you for showing me the Way, the Truth, and the Life. He reigns big in my heart. Your volunteering to be my folks, to be my friends. Your sacrifices for my betterment. You could have gotten distracted anywhere along the way with other things that wouldn't have looked "silly" in the world's eyes. Your square dancing friends back in the 60s. Your work friends in the 70s. Your bridge friends in the 80s. Thank you, thank you, thank you.

When Peter got out of the boat to go to Jesus, sinking, gulping water, Jesus stretched out His arm and caught Him. When they got into the boat and the sea calmed, the disciples worshipped Him. They praised Him. They were thanking Him. The first time in the Gospels that the disciples corporately showed Him their adoration. They had been saved!

That's it. Safe mode. That's how you can make all the "practices" of life. Now you know Dad's and my secret. Safe mode living bears all things, believes all things, hopes all things, endures all things. Safe mode living never fails. Although he didn't call it that, he lived it. All of it. He called it what most of you call it. He called it love. He had hideaways. He knew the worth of a person. He talked with Jesus. He said all his thank-yous.

American Airlines, the company that Mom worked for had a TV commercial back in the 1990s advertising *Miles for Kids*, kids who need transportation for special needs such as childhood cancer. The little girl says at the end of the commercial that she "can't wait to get up there again, where the sun is always shining and the sky is always blue." I can tell you, that's where Dad is. Where the Son—S O N—is always shining. Between the two operations that led up to his death, he was already raising his hands, praising his Lord. He made a deliberate effort to show us that. Now, eternally living in love. A "fisher come home."

Safe mode. It's available to everyone. It belongs on a mainframe though. The mainframe is Jesus. Accepting Him as your personal Lord and Savior is what Dad would have wanted for your life.

He had made the upgrade years ago.

Your love must come from Jesus.

This is how God showed his love among us: He sent his one and only Son into the world that we might live through him. This is love: not that we loved God, but that he loved us and sent his Son as an atoning sacrifice for our sins. Dear friends, since God so loved us, we also ought to love one another.
1 John 4:9-11

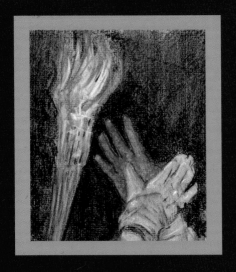

Neither a lofty degree of intelligence nor imagination nor both together go to the making of genius. Love, love, love, that is the soul of genius.
Wolfgang Amadeus Mozart

CHAPTER SIX

Not Always Calling the Play

Do all the good you can, by all the means
you can, in all the ways you can,
as long as ever you can.
John Wesley

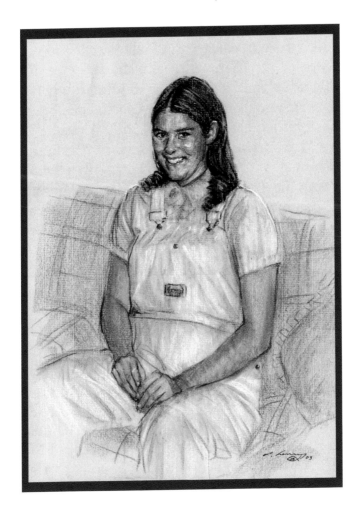

My first cousin, Molly (Wyatt) Strickler, was diagnosed with osteoblastoma of the thoracic spine, which differentiated to osteosarcoma and eventually took her precious life. Her disease progressed as my training in orthopaedic surgery and on into orthopaedic oncologic surgery progressed. I wish I had been involved. I can never get that opportunity back. Such is the chance that you have. You cannot reverse the course of time. The joy of helping or regret of not helping will stay with you forever.

We like to be in control, and when asked to help in the care of a patient with cancer, the situation is totally out of control it seems. Helping the person to the emergency room, to an unexpected doctor's visit, to an unanticipated need. Certainly someone closer to the person should be responsible. Certainly we are too busy and have lives and a family of our own. Certainly no one should expect us to put in another twenty hours a week on our already packed schedule. All those things take a back seat when the opportunity is gone. Believe me, I know.

A first cousin. A disease in my own field of expertise. Certainly I could have taken the time to visit her in the hospital, to consult with her treating physicians, to help explain the situation to her mother and father, my aunt and uncle. Don't make the same mistake I have made. Get involved.

Molly was a sweet young woman who held no remorse. Her trust was in Christ alone. Had I taken the time to be involved, I would have been the one blessed. As it is, I missed out on the blessing and actually had a negative impact by not taking the time. But don't get involved for the fear of the negative things that will ultimately occur (and they will). Get involved because you don't always have to call the play. You can listen to your heart's call and take the ball in that direction! You will be the stand out on the team. You will be the MVP.

Sometimes it is physically impossible to be of service. However, there is always the phone, the mail, e-mail, flowers, and the possibilities are endless. The ability to help is not always dependent upon the presence of the person. Don't let the possibility of spending money get you off the hook! A word of encouragement is much more needed in this instance than money. A word in love is always timely. And a listening ear is often enough for the time being.

And if you are a physician caring for those with cancer, take that extra time, the "uncoded time" to talk to a family member, a worried mother or father, about the strength that they may be lacking, the support that they may need. Caring for those with cancer is all about commitment to bring healing to the inner and the outer person, inseparable, yet both needing healing.

Make a commitment not to call the play, but to listen to the "Coach's voice," the voice of our Father in heaven. He is the caller of the play, and it is up to the players, us, to listen. We need to be reading His playbook, His Word, the Bible, in order to know the plays. Make a commitment to read God's Word to your friend or family member with cancer. Together you will both see the action unfold before you. You will understand the game plan, the blueprints, His design. You will be able to determine the outcome. What a wonderful number of memories you will gain of that person as you both reflect on His Word together.

You have the choice to choose whether to accept the love of Jesus.

We wait in hope for the Lord, he is our help and our shield. In him our hearts rejoice, for we trust in his holy name. May your unfailing love rest upon us, O Lord, even as we put our hope in you.
Psalm 33:20-22

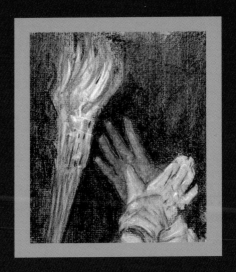

In the end, it is important to remember that we cannot become what we need to be by remaining what we are.
Max Depree

Not Taking the Shot

What we need . . . [is] love and wisdom
and compassion towards one another.
Robert Francis Kennedy

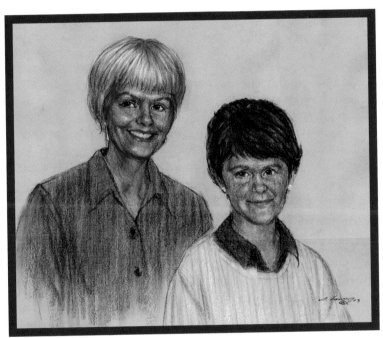

My mother's sister, Vera Crider, died of breast cancer at a young age. Her daughter, Christy Jan Mead, died of complications from diabetes and Hodgkin's lymphoma also at a young age. For a family to lose so much, it would be easy to become bitter and show resentment towards God and this life. Don't let that shot be taken. It only leads to defeat and broken relationships. I have never heard a discouraging word from Vera's other two children, Tom or Carrie, or from Christy's husband, Mark. Can you and I be that type of person? It doesn't come from what we're into, but what is into us.

Everyone is tempted to dwell on the disability and despair of living through cancer. We will, in all likelihood, be given another chance to help a friend or loved one through the challenges if we blow it this time. Take advantage of the situation to give your love away and if another occasion surfaces, you will be known as a giver of love. Not that it gets any easier or less challenging, but that it has become a *part* of you.

Trade the Sorrow

In Jeremiah 18, God is portrayed as the Potter, and we are the clay pots. If we are marred and thrown into the kiln of life, we will not be useful to hold the Living Water of life. If, however, we realize that what we are is inadequate for the situation, God can reshape us into useable vessels. It is what is inside of us as vessels that determines our worth. As I wrote this paragraph, during a tacet (not playing) for a piece titled *Trading the Sorrows* in an orchestra rehearsal for an Easter service, unknowingly I looked up to see a video of a potter's hands at work fade from the screen.

So it should be with your decision to be a vessel for others. Don't let your vessel be marred with bitterness or resentment. Move in God's Spirit. Let what you say be reflected by the "video" of your life. Let God fill your vessel with a gentle healing spirit. Let love flow from your spout! And let God be the pourer!

It has been my privilege to know those afflicted with cancer, to see their crises, and to often see their courage in their walk with their Lord, Jesus. I can remember Pedro, who through the Make-A-Wish Foundation, had his mother's home fixed up, not desiring the wish to be used on himself. A father of a Navajo boy with osteosarcoma who said to me that if he could, he would take the disease upon himself. The single mother who gave up her job to be devoted full time to her daughter with a malignancy of the pelvic bone. In my eyes, all these people have won over their disease. They have conquered part, if not all of cancer. They, with the help of a family member or friend like you, have prevailed in spirit and often physically as well. I have seen sorrow traded for joy. It has been a priceless experience.

You have only one life to give. Make it count. Give it to others. Give it to the one who has nothing to give in return. Give it to your loved one or friend with cancer. It will be a life filled with treasure. It will be a treasure that no one can steal and will never diminish in value no matter what the stock market or the world economy does. Jump in with both feet and be prepared to get wet!

You have the choice to choose whether to give the love of Jesus.

If I give all I possess to the poor and surrender my body to the flames, but have not love, I gain nothing. Love is patient, love is kind. It does not envy, it does not boast, it is not proud.
1 Corinthians 13:3-4

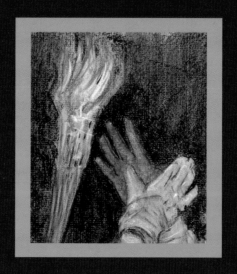

To know even one other life has breathed because you lived—this is to have succeeded.
Ralph Waldo Emerson

Not Seeing the Foul

Weakness is a better teacher than strength.
Mason Cooley

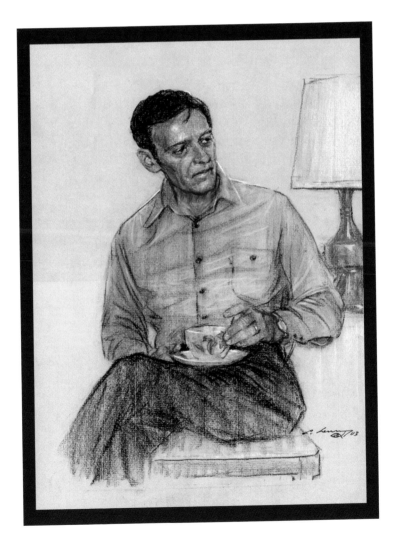

My father's brother, Edgar Roy Pitcher, Jr., my Uncle Eddie, was diagnosed with lung cancer while I was just starting orthopaedic oncologic surgery. He had been instrumental in the development of the infrared label scanner, although he was not given any of the credit. He didn't cry "foul" or seek to recover damages. He was a giving man, and even late in his life gave away many of the antique tools that he had collected and categorized. Was it because of his lifelong battle with the effects of childhood polio? He had learned not to see the foul.

I was asked to accept a generous gift to the Cancer Research and Treatment Center at the University of New Mexico from a group called the Odd Fellows. I had never heard of the organization but decided to talk to the group about what I thought an odd fellow is.

The Odd Fellow in Today's Society

Is an odd fellow a person who does an odd job? I certainly have an odd job, taking out huge pieces of people's bones and muscles and reconstructing them with titanium and cobalt chrome. I passed around two large metal knees used to reconstruct the knee and either the thigh bone or the leg bone. The group was mostly made up of older people and perhaps I had made a mistake saying I take out pieces of people but an older gentleman eagerly came up and took the prostheses. The fact is that is what I do. Not seeing the malignancy, the tumor is taken out without seeing it by taking out normal tissues

It got Mom, but it didn't *overtake* her. She, like Jesus saw the joy set before her. In Hebrews 12:1-2, the writer records, *"Therefore since we have so great a cloud of witnesses surrounding us, let us also lay aside every encumbrance, and the sin which so easily entangles us, and let us run with endurance the race that is set before us fixing our eyes on Jesus, the author and perfecter of faith, who for the joy set before Him endured the cross despising the shame, and set down at the right hand throne of God."* She showed me *the joy set before Jesus. That* is my most memorable memory of Mom.

Rob, Crystal, Wayne, Michael, John, Aaron, Rachel, whatever your name is, you are that joy also. Jesus died for you so that you may have abundant and everlasting life.

On the day of my mother's funeral, the Tulsa World's headline read, "Dandre goes home, 4 accused in custody." The 3-year-old boy "was found wandering the streets alone about 2 a.m. Monday in the 200 block of East 55th street North, a little more than 24 hours after his abduction. He had been feared dead. The boy was cold and wheezing when found. He was treated at a nearby hospital."

If there is anyone reading this, wandering the streets of life, honor Ann Pitcher on this day by accepting Jesus as your Lord and Savior. Talk to a pastor, a chaplain, or possibly your loved one's physician, or to me about accepting Him.

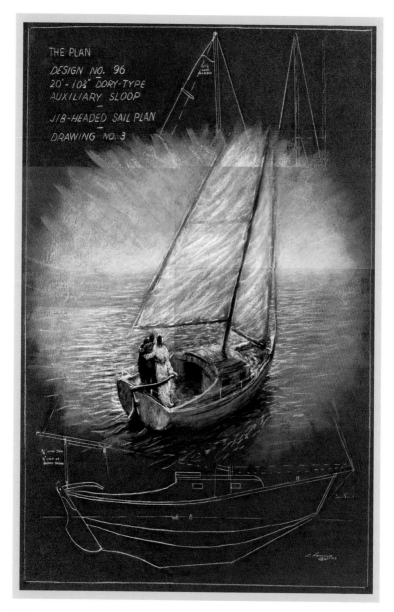

So what is my most memorable experience of Mom's life? Was it when she experienced Dad's death, or even her own? Both of those experiences, albeit painful, pointed me in the direction of my most memorable memory of Mom's life: *the joy set before Jesus.*

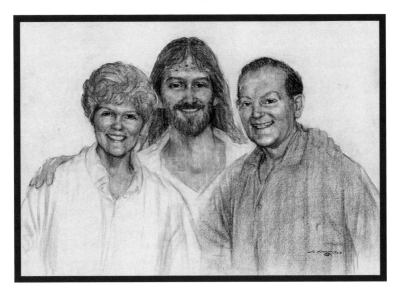

Jesus has taken away the absurdity of death and has made it a covered passageway for those who have accepted His blood sacrifice, atoning our lives. He did it for us. He did it because He saw us as the joy set before Him.

Mom showed me that all of you, of us, the joy set before Jesus, are my most memorable experience. People she loved, that is what Jesus' death was all about.

❖ ❖ ❖

And now you know from where the love comes.

*Be imitators of God, therefore, as dearly
loved children and live a life of love,
just as Christ loved us and gave
himself up for us as a fragrant
offering and sacrifice to God.*
Ephesians 5:1-2

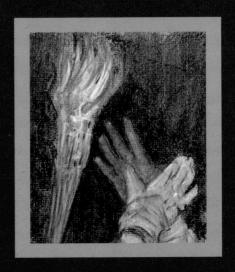

*The value of life lies not
in the length of days,
but in the use you make of them.*
Michel de Montaigne

CHAPTER ELEVEN

Not Getting the Credit

Action springs not from thought,
but from a readiness for responsibility.
Dietrich Bonhoeffer

The first person I treated who eventually died from his malignancy was Orville March. He had a malignancy called "malignant fibrous histiocytoma" of the thigh. It spread to his lungs despite radiation therapy, and despite chemotherapy he died. The surgical resection had been successful, but over a year later Orville died. I had the opportunity to take him to a dinner performance of *Scrooge, the Musical.* I considered him a real friend. It wasn't my involvement, but another patient of mine who made the real difference in his life. I can't remember his name, but in my mind, he gets the credit for helping Orville through his disease.

That may be what happens to you. You put in all this effort, and years from now, people forget your name. This must not be a concern for you. The brand names of the snowmobiles that carried my daughter, Crystal, and I to the top of Greenie Peak in northern New Mexico have long been forgotten! True love is not concerned with getting the credit. Nor does it ever stop, even when a loved one wins or loses a battle against cancer.

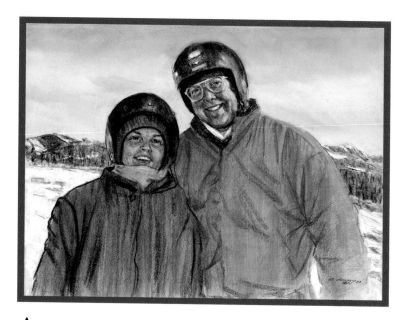

A patient of mine, Priscilla, became involved with enlisting bone marrow transplant donors. Another patient became involved in the "Make A Wish Foundation." Get involved in an organization making a difference in the lives of those living with cancer. Organize a cookie decorating party on Valentine's Day, volunteer at a Kids With Cancer Camp, bring "Meals On Wheels" to the hospice patient, donate your airline miles to those who need a flight for treatment, shave your head to help raise money for kids with cancer. There are as many ways to get involved as there are patients with cancer. And until we beat this dreadful and unfair disease, and beat it we will, there will be a need for your selfless love.

There are many lessons I've seen learned from supporting a person with cancer. First of all, suffering shows us *the love of the Father*. It was He who sent His own Son to die on the cross for our sins. It was He who said that He would suffer for us. And it is the one who truly loves another who says in his or her heart, that if he or she could, they would take the cancer and suffering upon themselves and give their lives for their loved one.

Second, it shows us *the longing of the Father*. He wishes to hold us in His arms, to give us His strength. His arm is not shortened, even in the face of a malignant diagnosis. Sometimes He calms the storm, and the malignancy is cured. Other times He calms His child, and we see His mighty strength as we could have never seen in another situation. Whatever the outcome, His desire is that we come to Him knowing that the outcome is in His control.

Finally, it shows us *the liberation of the Father*. Whether our loved one is healed, or goes to be with the Father, it is a time of celebration. Freed from the memories of the malignancy or from the worries of this world, he or she can be liberated from the chains of cancer.

It is an honor and a privilege to see the Father at work on behalf of His children. To hear that He finally has the full attention of a person. That He has given a firm acquittal of a person and that person is now walking by His side. That He has delivered a fathomless assurance that He will never forsake that person. The change in a person's life who offers his or herself as a servant to one who has cancer is unmistakably a miracle. A miracle in the face of calamity. A miracle which reaches beyond our own life and takes us to the heights we could not obtain otherwise.

❖   ❖   ❖

Give God the credit as the true love giver.

This is how we know what love is: Jesus Christ laid down his life for us.
And we ought to lay down our lives for our brothers.
1 John 3:16

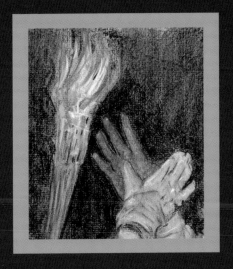

Only the heart knows how to find what is precious.
Fyodor Dostoyevsky

CHAPTER TWELVE

Not Giving Up

Go as far as you can see, and when
you get there you will see farther.
Elbert Hubbard

It seems intuitive that when a loved one dies, that is not the end of the pain. However, we as humans often take the easier road and withdraw from the person's or family's loss. People want their loved ones to be remembered, so don't stop recalling the moments of joy that person gave.

When all is said and done, we often feel that we have to have the answer to all the questions. Don't try to explain the circumstances, but be there to encourage and comfort. It's OK to say "I don't know." The journey with someone who has cancer is like climbing a previously unconquered mountain. It isn't going to be easy, and it is much easier to climb as a team. In today's hectic world however, we often find ourselves wanting only what we think is true joy and happiness.

Don't Avoid Spending Time with the Hurting

In 1994 my son, John, and I climbed Mount St. Helens in Washington. The climb up the 8,365 foot mountain was about a 4,000 vertical climb over a 4 mile trail. We went with orthopaedic residents from the Madigan

Army Medical Center residency program where I instructed at that time. All these young men were in superb shape. It was all I could do to keep up. John, who was only 12 at that time kept up until about 500 yards from the summit when he sat down on a boulder. I was nearing the summit and turned around to see where he was. He wasn't moving, but just sitting there, leaning on his pickax. To go back down or continue to reach the summit with the residents? That was the question. And I was tuckered out.

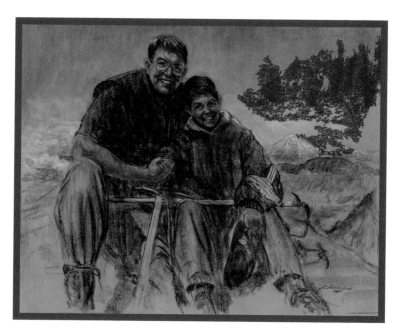

Don't Declare That You
"Understand" Because You Don't

I stumbled down the icy slope on my legs that felt like rubber. It was all I could do to keep from falling head first down the steep descent. I made it down to

John to see that he had been crying. "I can't make it," he managed to get out. I sat down beside him, completely worn out, out of breath, and not looking forward to getting back on the ascent and said, "I'm not sure I can either." We both looked into each other's eyes, saw the agony, embraced in a big hug, got back up and made the rest of the climb!

At the funeral of a first cousin of mine, Christy Jan Mead, who lost her life from complications of diabetes and Hodgkin's lymphoma at the age of forty-seven, her husband Mark and two young children, Matthew and Yanna sat in the front pew during the memorial service. I was so blessed by their testimonies of their wife and mother's life. Tears flowed down my cheeks when I listened to the words the thirteen-year-old Matthew had written. I don't understand all the ramifications of a diagnosis of malignancy or even death in this world, but I do know that they both can be a time when families are drawn together. They can be a time of healing.

Don't Offer, "Just Call if You Need Anything at All"

A hurting person won't call. God is preparing you and me. We must share the character of God which is to reach those who need us. To outstretch our hands to them. You will gain much more than you give in return. It will be evident of where your love comes from and where your love is taking you. In Hebrews 2:10 we read, "*In bringing many sons to glory, it was fitting that God, for whom and through whom everything exists, should make the author of their salvation perfect through suffering.*" As you give Christ Jesus' love, you are becoming more like Him.

Don't Just Believe That the Pain Will Simply Go Away

Pain of living with cancer is deeper than the bone. It is the pain of the thought of leaving those we love. The fear of what lies ahead. The follow-up surveillance studies that may indicate a relapse. The doctors' visits. The lab tests. The imaging studies. What may be around the next corner may add to the pain. It is all unknown.

It is a mystery to me why some people are healed and some are not. Jesus Himself has carried our sicknesses and pain, yet it seems that some of our prayers are unanswered. Seeing outside the human "box" is a characteristic of love. Knowing that God is in control is its feature that sets it apart from human nature. Sometimes the pain is not so much severe as sustained. A mild pain that is constant can be as draining as an intermittent severe pain. Being there during the pain can be a painful and draining experience. Only sustained by Jesus' love will you be a pain reliever for your loved one.

Don't Ever Give Up

I have had patients who wish to never die, those who wish to have as much time as possible, and those who wish to die quickly and be done quickly as not to be a burden to anybody. It is not up to you to decide what your friend or loved one should decide for his or her life, but to be there to show your love and support for their decisions. Let them know that you respect and support their choices. Encourage them to seek God's love through His Word, the Bible. Read to them. Listen to them. Hold them in His love.

When the nights are long, the days are cold, be with them. It is an act of courage and a shield against discouragement. It says that "you matter to me." Other people may or may not be watching, but rest assured, God sees your selflessness. He never has given up on us. Let's pass it on. . . .

Learning how to give Christ Jesus' love to others is the purpose of life; never, never, never ever give up.

Dear friends, let us love one another, for love comes from God. Everyone who loves has been born of God and knows God. Whoever does not love does not know God, because God is love. This is how God showed his love among us: He sent his one and only Son into the world that we might live through him. This is love: not that we loved God, but that he loved us and sent his Son as an atoning sacrifice for our sins. Dear friends, since God so loved us, we also ought to love one another.
1 John 4:7-12

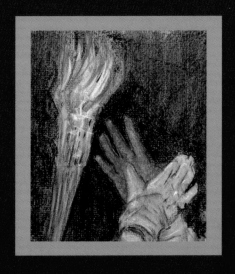

Service is the rent we pay for being . . . not something you do in your spare time.
Marion Wright Edelman

Not Missing the Postgame Show

by Ingrid Sharon, MD
Breast Surgeon
Colorado Springs, Colorado

The measure of a life, after all,
is not its duration, but its donation.
Corrie Ten Boom

We have more in common with those for whom we are caring than we think. We are all one day closer than we were yesterday to meeting God. Confronted by their mortality, some of them are preparing for that day. Are you and I?

As Dr. Pitcher said, God put skin on and came in the flesh as Jesus the Messiah. He lived a perfect life, and thereby gained the right to take the blame and punishment for every wrong thing we ever thought or did. The wages of sin is death, the Bible says. Jesus died in our place. If we place our trust in Him, we can have eternal life with Him and the others who have chosen Him. That means that our loved ones who believe in Him are not "gone." They have only "gone ahead." It is not "good-bye," but rather, "see you later."

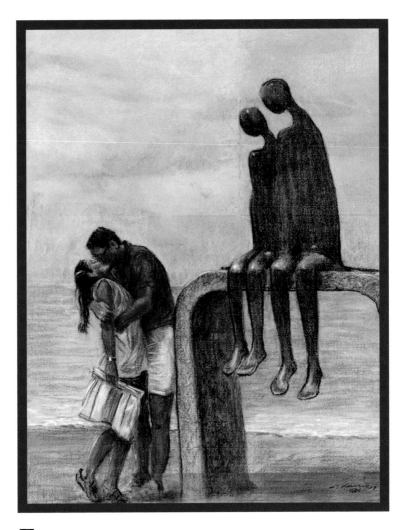

Everything in this life is temporary (my father taught me that). Even this temporal physical life. We get to take one thing to heaven with us, though: our relationships. So invest in people. God did. Be like Him. Give your time, help, gifts, love to people . . . because people last forever.

Jesus said He would give the Holy Spirit to those who ask . . . we ask for bread, fish, healing . . . God answers many times just by giving more of Himself, His Holy Spirit. He Himself is the ultimate answer to our questions: His presence with us, Emmanuel. He is Jehovah Shammah, the God who is there. Be like God. Be there for people.

Jesus said we have not because we ask not. So ask what your loved one wants so you know how to pray. The young mother of four asked that her seventeen month old would remember her as "Mom." The divorcing woman asked that her husband would reconcile, preferring to be widowed to being divorced. The estranged sister asked that her brother would go on a final trip with her. I admit I also usually ask for a miracle . . . because I never want to learn that my patient missed out on a miraculous healing because I did not ask.

The latter rain is coming. Be a part of it by making yourself available to God for His purposes for your life. Love Him. Obey Him. Be holy. Go forth and dispense His hope. He is the God of hope. Hope is the target at which faith aims. God is love. Make the abundant glorious display of His love through you the aim of your life as you walk alongside your loved one going through the chapter in their life called "cancer."

Giving Christ's love to others as if it were your last measure of devotion will be a glorious display of His love; it will influence others towards His holiness and saving grace.

Now that you have purified yourselves by obeying the truth so that you have sincere love for your brothers, love one another deeply, from the heart.
1 Peter 1:22

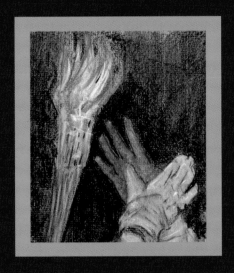

We make a living by what we get, but we make a life by what we give.
Winston Churchill

Not Missing the Locker Room Celebration

There are only two options regarding commitment. You're either in or out. There's no such thing as a life in-between.
Pat Riley

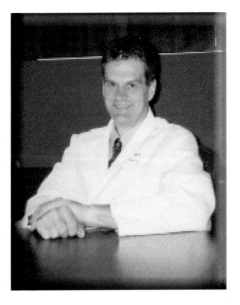

H. Thomas Temple, MD, is an orthopaedic oncologic surgeon at the University of Miami and Director of the Miami Tissue Bank and the orthopaedic Oncologic Division. He received his training at Walter Reed Army Medical Center in Washington D.C., and his orthopaedic oncologic surgery fellowship at the Combined Harvard orthopaedic Program at Massachusetts General Hospital and The Children's Hospital in Boston, Massachusetts.

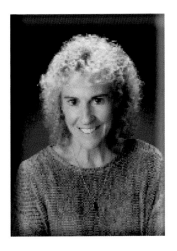

Sue Hefflefinger is a speech/language pathologist in the Albuquerque Public School system who found herself caring for her husband, Steve, when he was diagnosed with Hodgkin's lymphoma. It is people like her who have inspired the writing of this book.

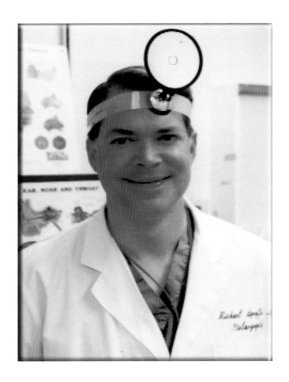

Michael Spafford, MD, is a head and neck oncologic surgeon at The University of New Mexico and the New Mexico Veterans Administration Health Care System. He is board certified in otolaryngology and is an avid Christian. He completed a residency in otolaryngology at the University of Colorado in Denver and a fellowship in head and neck oncologic surgery at the Johns Hopkins University Kimmel Cancer Center.

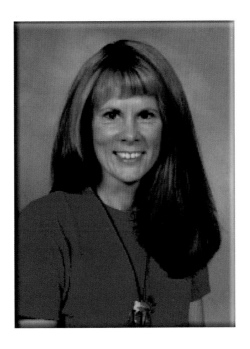

Ingrid Sharon, MD, was a medical school classmate of Dr. Pitcher's from 1978 until 1982. She now is a breast surgical oncologist practicing in Colorado Springs, Colorado. She is a member of the American Society of Breast Surgeons. She loves her patients and has devoted her life to show them daily the love of Jesus. She says that she will be unemployed when she reaches heaven, but taking classes in remedial reading classes to replace her current vocabulary of "cancer, pain, paresthesias, infection, bleeding. . . ." It is evident from her life that important words such as hope, care, and love, are already in her thesaurus.

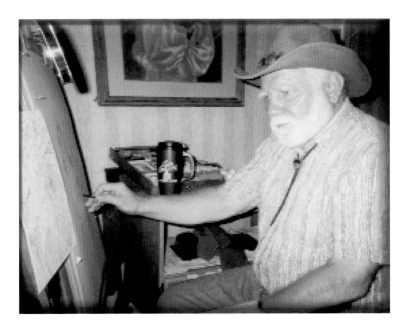

L. Henry (Hank) Jones was born in Ferriday, Louisiana, finished high school in Cleveland, Mississippi, and attended the University of Auburn in Alabama. After a four-year hitch in the Navy he graduated from the University of New Mexico, and spent a few years in the commercial art field before he set up shop in 1971 as a full-time portrait artist. Since that time he has completed over twenty thousand portrait commissions in addition to many depictions of the Southwest. He works from "live" sittings, but a good portion of his work is done from photos. His favorite medium is pastel. His artist wife, Jovenia, and he have three children, one who has gone to be with the Lord. They live in Albuquerque where they maintain a studio in their home. He is willing to share his love for Jesus with whoever God places in the chair in front of him.

J. David Pitcher, Jr., MD
University of Miami School of Medicine
Department of Orthopaedics
P.O. Box 016960 (D-27)
Miami, Florida 33101

Involve other people in the
chapters of your life . . .